The ~~Perfect~~ Couple

The Ultimate Guide to a Fulfilling Marriage for Newlyweds

Monica B. Jackson

Terms and Conditions

LEGAL NOTICE

The Publisher has strived to be as accurate and complete as possible in the creation of this report, notwithstanding the fact that he does not warrant or represent at any time that the contents within are accurate due to the rapidly changing nature of the Internet.

While all attempts have been made to verify information provided in this publication, the Publisher assumes no responsibility for errors, omissions, or contrary interpretation of the subject matter herein. Any perceived slights of specific persons, peoples, or organizations are unintentional.

In practical advice books, like anything else in life, there are no guarantees of income made. Readers are cautioned to reply on their own judgment about their individual circumstances to act accordingly.

This book is not intended for use as a source of legal, business, accounting or financial advice. All readers are advised to seek services of competent professionals in legal, business, accounting and finance fields.

You are encouraged to print this book for easy reading.

Table Of Contents

FOREWORD

CHAPTER 1
Introduction
The Basic

CHAPTER 2
Marriage And Survival
Surviving

CHAPTER 3
Problems With The First Marriage
Hardships
Expectations
Intimacy
Connection
Money

CHAPTER 4
Potential Remedies For Marital Issues
Solutions

CHAPTER 5
Education For Early Marriages
Education

CHAPTER 6
The Fundamental Soft Skills For Newlyweds
Skills
Love
How to prepare
Communication

CHAPTER 7

Hard Talents That Newlywed Couples Must Possess

Strong Skills

Finding Solutions

Prioritizing Your Spouse

Be A Forgiver

Chapter 8

The Advantages Of Maintaining A Marriage

Advantages

Being Content With Life

Safeguarding Your Kids

Become Financially Stable

CHAPTER 9

The A-Z Of Marital Advice

Tips

Advice

Devotion

Honesty

Intimacy

Laughter

Parenting

CONCLUSION

The Long-Term Remedies For Marital Issues

FOREWORD

It may be challenging to make it through the first year of marriage when you are a new couple, particularly if you are still getting to know one another. Generally, getting to know someone before getting married is preferable, but we all know this isn't how real life works. You meet someone wonderful who instantly warms your heart, and before you realize it, you're in love. You've already been thinking about getting married for some time and jumping right in. Couples from all over the globe have shown it many times previously. Learn all you need right here.

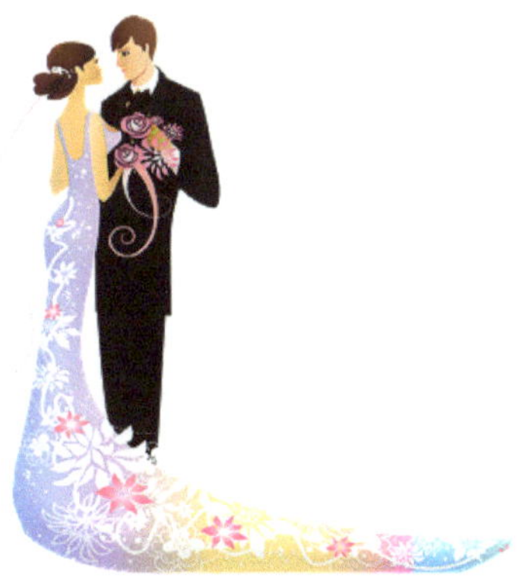

Survival Of A First-Year Marriage
How New Couples Can Survive Their First Year
of Marriage

CHAPTER 1
Introduction

If the two of you haven't even shared a home yet, there's a significant possibility that after you move in together, disagreements will start to happen. This is something that often occurs in various circumstances. In reality, it's the "stages" of your relationship.

Every relationship passes through different phases regardless of how close you are to the other person. Your spouse may just put his trash wherever he is standing, but you may be a fussy person who likes things to be pristine.

Other concerns might include when to be intimate when to work late, when to go out with friends, and how you manage housework. All of these factors might affect how well you two get along. Rules should be set up so that you two may have a happy marriage.

The Basic

Marriage is more than simply a means of survival. The significance is deeper than that. Making sacrifices for the person you genuinely love is a key component of marriage.

You take time off work to care for them while they are ill. Give your lover more of your time if they are angry that you are going out a lot and not paying attention to them. Making minor changes may make a significant difference and lessen the intensity of disputes in the relationship.

Never take your partner for granted; make sure they know how much they mean to you daily. Because you never know when you'll run into them again, it's crucial.

One of the most crucial components of marriage is communication. The relationship will fail if you can't talk to your spouse. Attempt to speak less and listen more. Or, if you tend to speak more than you listen, it's time to listen to them. Perhaps your partner wants you to pay attention to them so you can fully understand their perspective on a certain issue.

CHAPTER 2

Marriage And Survival

You must first be aware of your priorities if you want to endure marriage. Despite what your parents may advise, work should never be your priority. Always put your marriage first. After all, they are the one who lives in the same house as you, prepares meals, earns more income for the two of you, assists with child care, and sometimes engages in intimate behavior.

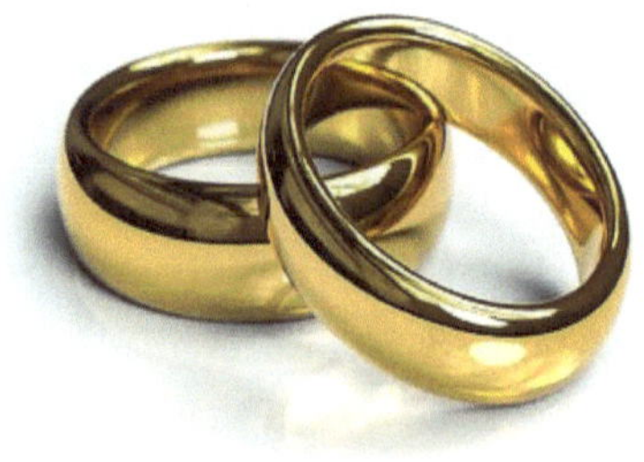

Surviving

There are many things to accomplish in a marriage, and in this day and age, most couples work together. Men aren't accustomed to doing tasks that a woman would perform, making marriage challenging. For instance, most men object to cleaning the bathroom or ironing their clothes. They really wouldn't do anything like that. Also, don't bother growing flowers in the backyard. Even the blossoms are beyond their reach.

Fathers instill in their sons a desire to work hard and get a solid education to support their families. They cannot get pregnant or develop a deep bond with their kid. Usually, the mother's emotional state increases after giving the baby. For a guy to accept the truth, they must see his kid. They expect us to care for everything around the home and do not comprehend what pregnant women go through.

Women tend to be more emotional and chat more than they do housework. Guess who they contact if the toilet leaks or the sink is broken? They panic and contact their spouse. The women excel in household tasks like cooking great meals, folding clothes, and getting ready for the dance their husband is taking them to after work.

Both the guy and the lady are sleeping in the same bed. The lady is reading her book, paying close attention to what she reading. The only thing a guy can think about is intimate sexual relations. He starts talking to her at this point, even attempting to massage her.

It works and doesn't work sometimes. When males succeed, they often advance to the top and carry out their duties. Their spouse then just lays there while attempting to regain her breath.

The guy already nods to sleep without expressing affection or any other kind of gratitude. It's as though nothing ever occurred. This is the case since most guys are emotionless and act as they choose.

It might be difficult to divide daily tasks and attempt to engage in emotional or physical contact. Right now, this is the reason why marriages are ending in divorce. They cannot communicate effectively with and treat their partner fairly. All it takes is collaboration, listening, and empathy when it comes to the other person.

CHAPTER 3

Problems With The First Marriage

When it comes to marriage, there are several challenges. Expectations, closeness, connection, and money are the most common. Each of these subjects has the potential to cause issues. The woman may get angry and just want her husband to quit spending a lot of money on his gaming activities. They need that cash for their kids.

The lady is yet another illustration. She is often preoccupied with household chores and feels stressed out, making sex the last thing on her mind. The husband enjoys intimacy very much, but without it, he could feel like he is drifting away from his wife.

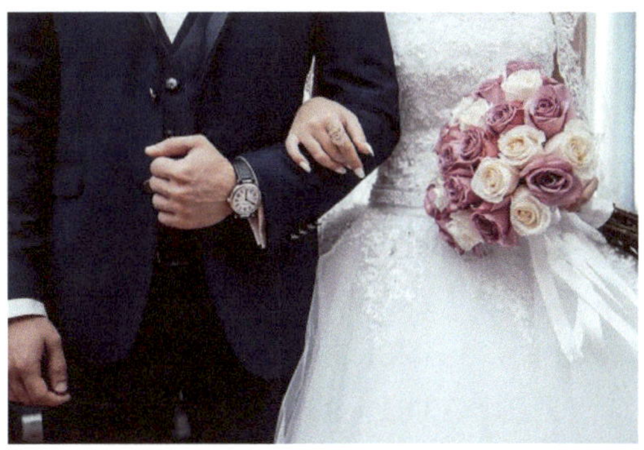

Hardships

You know, it takes a lot of tiny things to spark a fight between a husband and wife. They can harbor resentment towards one another and be unable to resolve their differences. The other person may try, but there are instances when they aren't as cooperative as they are. This is why relationships are so challenging. Here are the four challenges that marriage presents:

Expectations

When you go home, the wife has such high hopes for you. She forbids you from eating in your room because she thinks there could be crumbs on the bed. She also doesn't want you to leave your towel on the floor. You're not at all excited about this. On the other hand, you anticipate that your wife will always be dressed to the nines and ready for supper when you get home. You only actually care about this.

Intimacy

It's crucial to comprehend how your spouse feels if he's too exhausted to do anything with you even though you've been seeking intimacy for a few weeks. Give him a gentle back rub to show him that you care rather than exert pressure. He could be dealing with a lot of stress at work. It is true for both men and women when it comes to intimacy.

Connection

Making a connection with your other half is crucial. There is no place for divorce or a breakup if you share a strong bond. Most connected couples often have a greater understanding of one another. In a relationship, empathy and sympathy go hand in hand. They are depressed if their companion is. Depending on how long a couple has been together, it might sometimes take a few years or less than a few months for them to feel completely attached.

Money

Sadly, one of the main causes of divorce is financial problems. Your relationship will suffer if you struggle with money management and bills build up often. It is stretched due to the tension brought on by financial troubles.

CHAPTER 4
Potential Remedies For Marital Issues

The advantages of being married are many, and your marriage will strengthen if you stick together to resolve issues as they come. Remember that you'll both want to work on your marriage's issues.

It will only be a one-way street if one person is prepared to seek treatment or speak to you about the problems in the marriage. This indicates that there will be no advancement in the marriage.

It's crucial to explain to your partner why you want certain marital practices to change. Inform them that you are serious and may file for divorce if they don't change.

When your spouse notices that you are doing business, they may wish to modify some of their routines. Of course - don't be shocked if they discuss part of what you do when the two of you sit down. They may also talk to you about your negative tendencies regarding marriage, which is acceptable.

Solutions

Finding answers is relatively simple in a marriage, but adhering to them isn't always simple. You two must overcome this, and communication is essential if one of you struggles to stay committed to your objectives.

The other person may see their error and admit that, despite their best efforts, they are powerless to change. Some individuals are at a stage when they don't want to change. They must be motivated to change by something. Most of the time, they want to retain you and improve their family life.

You should be aware that not all your suggestions for potential marital solutions will succeed. For instance, your wife could even urge you to borrow money if you establish separate bank accounts due to her spending tendencies. Because you can see her behaviors returning, this stresses the marriage and might result in arguments.

Perhaps this time, it's not the wife. Your spouse often leaves you at home as he goes to obscene strip clubs. He argues that you have never had sexual relations with him.

Tell him that doing this is unacceptable and that you should take a few days off if he persists in doing it. When you get back, concentrate on your relationship's closeness. Are you too worn out for intimacy?

Him? Before you both go to bed, pay attention to his requirements. Don't make it seem like a job; make it enjoyable. We guess that when you two initially started dating, you both found enjoyment in one another. He will respect you and come home more regularly if you bring him back to this period. If he doesn't, it may be best to move on, as this wasn't truly his reason for leaving.

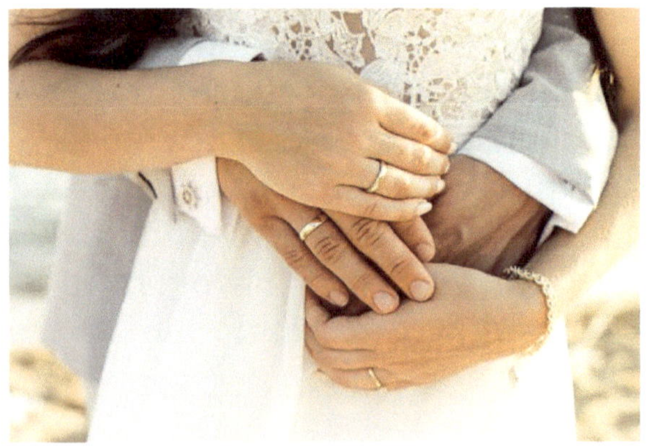

CHAPTER 5
Education For Early Marriages

Do you know what kind of schooling is available for young marriages? There are about five phases of a marriage when the couple learns to know one another, encounters difficulties, disagrees, resolves these difficulties, focuses on their children, and succeeds in their union.

In most cases, this will take several years. Some couples, though, are fortunate from the beginning. They have known one other for so long that they are familiar with each other's behaviors and no longer need to work on their marriage. Everything appears to spontaneously spring to life. It is clear how intimately attached the two of you are when this occurs.

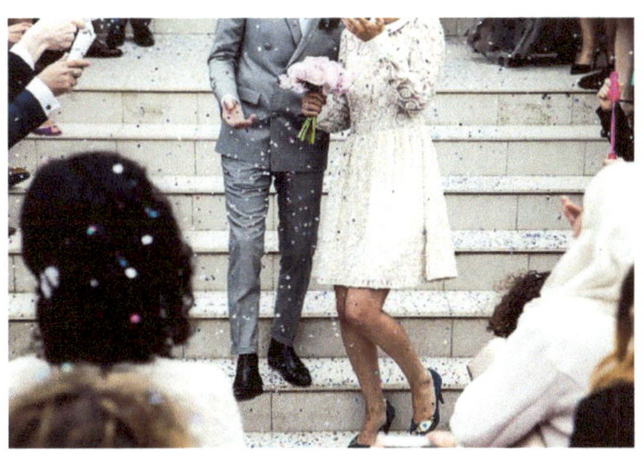

Education

If you have relationship issues, you could be in the beginning stages of "reality." You are just now beginning to understand how they behave in various circumstances. When your spouse is furious or agitated, you could witness them at their worst. It might be frightening when your spouse displays these kinds of feelings for the first time. This often results in disputes in the future.

Let's examine some of the early marriage education options and how each stage plays out: The honeymoon period is when a couple is often most enthusiastic about one another, and the romance appears to start on its own. This is because their lives are going well for them. Most couples enjoy romantic moments as well as enjoyable sexual activities with one another. Couples go out to eat, work together, and attend events during this time. Either before or after their wedding, they might enter the honeymoon period. The answer mostly relies on how long you've known the individual.

Reality Stage: During this phase, some couples experience a sense of loss and even start comparing one another to a former lover. They start to think they are incompatible with that individual and that the relationship is a mistake. Sadness, disillusionment, and even rage may manifest. This is quite natural, and couples go through it because issues are about to worsen.

Through. When a couple is close to one another, they often notice the person's "poor" traits. The other party feels devastated by this and isn't sure what to do about the relationship. Almost always, The reality stage often lasts up to two years.

Family Stage: Due to certain potential tensions, the relationships become closer throughout the childbearing years. Everything is geared around the children rather than the marriage itself. Instead of going on a romantic date, the guy and lady put in more effort to achieve their objectives. They understand how much planning goes into raising a family.

After they have a kid together, they will grow even closer because they want to do everything they can to make their child happy. When the reality period has passed, you both will know how to manage concerns like the baby crying, medical visits, and financial difficulties that may come now.

The success stage—If you have been married for ten years or more, you have probably already passed this stage. Usually, by the time your kids are teenagers or adults, you've already experienced every possible marital hardship. It is reasonable to conclude that you have discovered a life mate with whom you will be together till death. Congratulations!

CHAPTER 6

The Fundamental Soft Skills For Newlyweds

Are you recently wed and curious about the fundamental soft skills you'll need to succeed in your marriage? You cannot expect too much from your spouse to do this, and communication is essential. Accepting your spouse for who they are and how they act is crucial.

Any negative behaviors or habits may always be discussed later, but wait until therapy. It's best for the two of you to quarrel sometimes and learn to live with your irritating in-laws. If there are many issues, you may deal with them all at once.

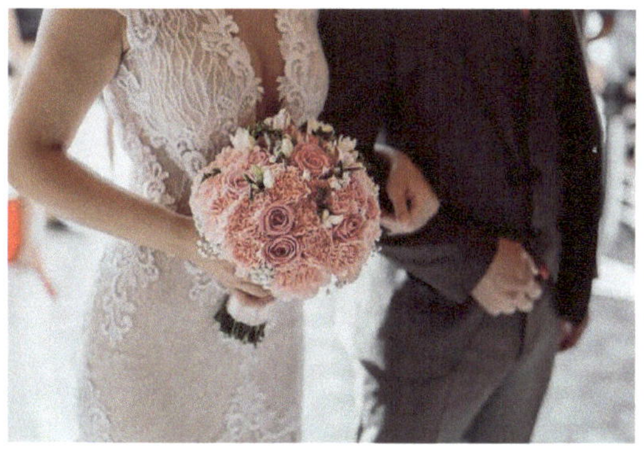

Skills

Love

Unconditional love for the other person is the main factor in a relationship. There is a significant possibility that the two of you will succeed if you love them for who they are rather than how they seem. It's possible that your wife, who is now really attractive, may later get larger due to the past two children she gave you.

In a different scenario, even if you like your attractive spouse dearly, something has altered his circumstances. Recently, a bear mauled him, leaving him with several scars.

The two of you became closer, and despite his facial scars and some deformities, you still like him for who he is as a person. He's always been a hilarious, gregarious person. Love him deeply, and be grateful that he's still here. Remember that the assault may have been deadly if it had been serious enough.

How to prepare

Whatever you do, avoid bugging your spouse or having high expectations for them. For them, this could be quite distressing. At this time, it is preferable to support them and provide advice.

You will assist them in becoming better people and forming better habits by doing this. If your man was disorganized before you ever met him, there may

Have been a few minor adjustments. He picks up his coat rather than toss it on the ground. This is a sign of improvement, but don't anticipate him doing the dishes or the washing.

Communication

It's crucial to talk to your partner. Consider the marriage finished if you cannot address significant topics, difficulties, or dates in your relationship.

In this situation, you may still be in the reality phase of your marriage and are just now learning that your spouse is quite reserved among others. Give him a little nudge if he tends to be reserved with you.

You'll need to engage him in conversation and engage him in conversation by asking him questions. Try not to worry too much about it since he'll change his mind in time.

CHAPTER 7
Hard Talents That Newlywed Couples Must Possess

Although combining hard skills into a new marriage might be challenging, marriage can be lovely. However, you must take this action to guarantee that your marriage advances. If you don't, your marriage will end in divorce, leaving you with almost nothing.

Remember that family memories make up most of our lives and that Earth was created so that people may connect with one another. For us, this is priceless.

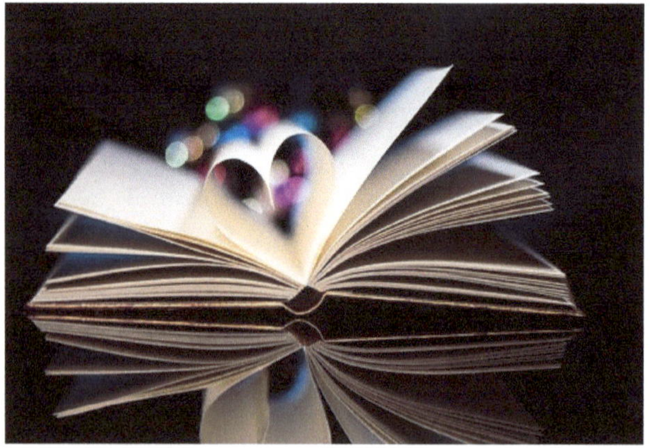

Instead of going out with friends, working too

much, or becoming stressed about little issues that have no bearing on the relationship, the family should always come first. Take your time and go slowly. Be firm with your spouse by bringing hard talents into the union. You should educate yourself on the following few:

Strong Skills

Finding Solutions

It is a continual struggle whenever the two of you want to go out to eat. He likes South American cuisine, while you just prefer sushi. He abhors sushi and doesn't care for anything that has fish or soy sauce on the side of the rice. When it's time to eat out, this makes you unhappy.

Consider going to two separate eateries to satisfy your respective cravings. You may prepare a romantic supper in the park or order takeout and enjoy it there. But if you want to dine at a genuine restaurant, simply bring your meal from the other restaurant. With this method, you will be content and stop fighting. As you can see, resolving conflicts in a marriage is crucial.

Prioritizing Your Spouse

Because most people are selfish, this is perhaps the hardest thing to accomplish. However, you should do this for your partner if you love them. Learn what they want.

You can always find space for your requirements another day. Speak with them if they are feeling anxious, depressed, or angry. Ask your partner if there is anything you can do to help them feel better. They'll begin to regard you with greater respect.

Be A Forgiver

In partnerships, the wife or husband often does something incorrectly and annoys the other person. Feelings of disappointment, rage, despair or even grief remain as a result.

Keep your emotions in check and ask them why they did what they did. You need to know why they treated you this way if cheating is a problem. When individuals cheat, it's often because their partner isn't meeting their needs.

Lack of emotional connection or intimacy is the most obvious cause. Depending on the marital issues, people may have an emotional or physical affair. Simply express to them how wounded you are and want to make it work instead of becoming angry. Allow them at least one more opportunity.

Chapter 8
The Advantages Of Maintaining A Marriage

For couples, surviving marriage offers several advantages. Some of these include developing personally, being more affectionate, communicating concerns to your spouse, and even achieving financial stability while working.

Marriage vows call for a lifetime commitment, and you should always be there for your partner. You will achieve mental wellness by doing this, and you will also benefit them.

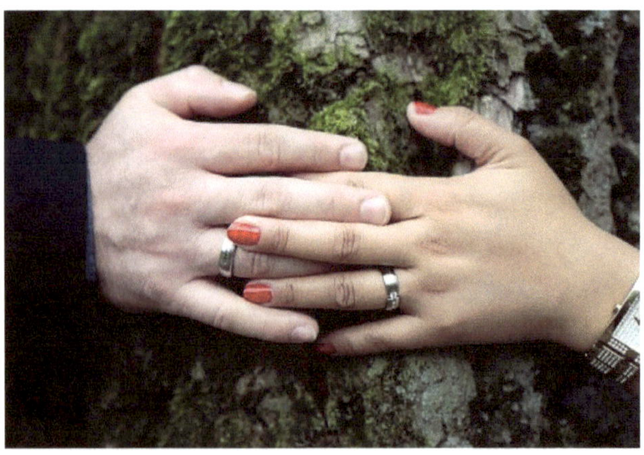

Given the damage that anger does to children when parents split, it is clear that your marriage will benefit your children. Do yourself a favor and save them from this ordeal. The greatest thing for your future is to take your time and make it work. Never give up!

Following are a few advantages of maintaining a marriage:

Advantages

Being Content With Life

You'll be a happier person in life when you're with someone you love. After all, friends are there to participate in your fun, lift your spirits, or be by your side through difficult moments. You may worry if you often attend the cancer hospital, but if your spouse is there to support you, your day will be a lot better. This is but one illustration of what we are referring to. If you have a companion, you won't have to deal with some circumstances alone. Unfortunately, some newly bereaved or divorced individuals are resentful and unkind toward others.

Safeguarding Your Kids

You are defending your kids by maintaining your marriage. For instance, many girls without dads are more prone to get pregnant early or adopt a rebellious attitude that may lead to drug or alcohol usage. A father's role is to safeguard his daughter from danger and to provide his daughter with love and discipline.

Additionally, some children experience sadness due to their parent's divorce. You'll want to check on our kids since they are so priceless. A parent may fall apart if they see their child grow up with anguish in their heart. We often go above and above to make our children happy.

Become Financially Stable

A household often requires the assistance of two persons. The situation is much worse if you have children. Due to unexpected medical visits, child-related expenses, and bill payments, a single mother who works only one job may be unable to make it through the month. Due to her financial difficulties, she could potentially be ejected from the house. However, you will achieve financial stability if two persons are employed. The two of you will be OK if you both manage your finances responsibly and pay your payments on time.

Check your bank account statements often to check what's happening and ensure your spouse doesn't have a problem with gambling. Money might "disappear" at any time. Identity theft or your spouse stealing money from you due to careless spending habits might be the cause of this. Only after you have been together for a few years and trust your partner should you open a joint bank account.

CHAPTER 9
The A-Z Of Marital Advice

Here are the A-Z marriage secrets and advice for newlyweds on how to have a happy marriage.

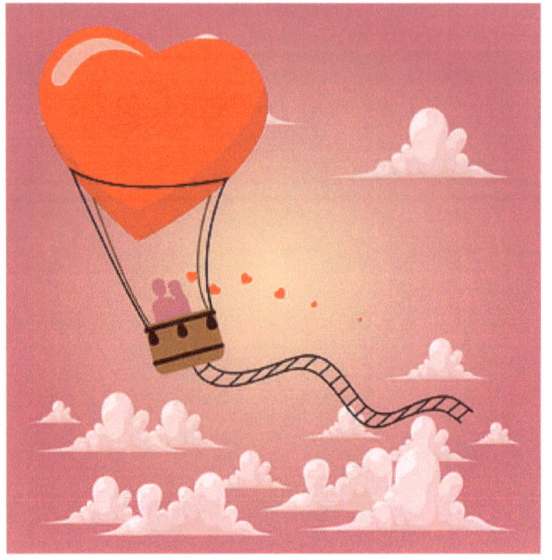

Tips

Advice

A fantastic technique to make the marriage function is giving your spouse advice when they are stressed or experiencing issues. They often won't vent their frustrations on you. Instead, they will feel compelled to be vulnerable and discuss their issues. The fact that your spouse is with you will be appreciated if you can provide them guidance. Not sure how to provide advice? No issue. You may simply hold them and give them a back rub. To give the impression that you are concerned about their difficulties, ask them additional questions regarding the situation. Most guys don't want to hear about every minute of their wife's day. A few details are acceptable, but if you give them too much, they can feel overwhelmed and lose words.

Devotion

Making date evenings happen, seeing your spouse often, and making time for them even when you're busy are all signs of dedication to your mate. Go for it if you have a brief opportunity to spend time with them on your day off! Visit your loved one often if they are in the hospital and haven't been able to walk for a month. Bring flowers for them and let them know how much you care. By demonstrating your commitment, you'll let them understand how much you value them, and they'll form a close relationship with you. These connections will develop into something more and often continue for many years.

Honesty

If you are already trustworthy, this can be simple for you. Did everyone at your crazy party decide it would be humorous to doodle on your white wall at home? Even when you arrived home, you were unaware that this had occurred. Your spouse informed you that the person who painted the walls was your son. However, your son was at the event and using a toy camera to take photographs. Remember that this camera produces films for children. You are upset about what your spouse did after discovering all the photos.

As you can see, honesty improves the relationship even when it is your fault. If you can't trust someone in a relationship, you'll always analyze their every move. Neither you nor your spouse is in good health if you do this. You don't want to point out any wrongdoing on their part. Perhaps they did nothing wrong, and you are the one who has to apologize to them. See what transpires when there is a lack of honesty in the relationship? It just makes matters worse.

Intimacy

Did you know that love and intimacy go hand in hand? Men will see sexual closeness in the bed as a type of love, even though some women may disagree. They feel it is therapeutic in a sexual way. After having sex with their spouses, most men get closer to them. Additionally, foreplay is crucial for women. Men should be aware of this, also. Your wife can think that you don't value or cherish her body if you hurry this with her. Enjoy yourself and take your time. You'll have a better time overall.

Laughter

Sharing a laugh with your spouse is enjoyable and encourages you to "play" together. Do you recall pushing your spouse into the pool while he was still covered? At the moment, he wasn't pleased, but you both subsequently laughed about it. The images you captured of him looking shocked and falling were hilarious. He couldn't help but chuckle at what had transpired. Tickling or making fun of one another is a surefire way to make someone smile. You are making lifelong memories every time the two of you laugh together. You are shoving anything negative in your life away by laughing. Another method of healing is through laughter.

Parenting

It's crucial to be a good parent to your kids. Your marriage is impacted by how you treat your kids. Likely, you sometimes shout at the kids if you're a stressed-out mother whose children won't listen to you. Your spouse disapproves of this since he is highly composed and sympathetic. Analyze his behavior when the kids are misbehaving to discover what dad does. Learn from him or parenting books. How you raise your children will impact them for the rest of your life, and, believe it or not, your actions impact people around you.

CONCLUSION

The Long-Term Remedies For Marital Issues

You'll need to start problem-solving to discover long-lasting answers for your marriage. Every marital issue, including money, adultery, parenting, and so on, ought to have a remedy. Here are some long-term remedies to help you stay married:

Concentrate On Yourself

This strategy, believe it or not, is effective. Find out what about you irritate your spouse, then focus on that aspect of yourself. If they claim you are being too overpowering, try to remain cool. Practice mind-clearing techniques and develop your independence. You are putting yourself in a better relationship by doing this. You can do most of the work without depending on what he or she performs.

Limit your expectations

Your partner will become unhappy in the relationship if you have unreasonable expectations of them. They could harbor resentment against you, leading to dishonesty, disputes, or even a creeping withdrawal from you.

Consult a counselor

Speaking with a counselor is preferable to battling about trivial issues. You won't have to worry about this conversation becoming an argument since both sides can be heard. The counselor will be able to discuss some of the progress the couple has made together, and things may improve from where they were.